"..Barbara por Atras"
A Latin Woman's Guide to Fitness

Barbara Trujillo Gomez
with Blanca Rodríguez

B&B Fit, LLC

For further information, please visit:
barbaraporatras.com

Printed in Canada

"...Barbara por Atras": A Latin Woman's Guide to Fitness
Barbara Trujillo Gomez with Blanca Rodríguez

1. Title 2. Author 3. Fitness

Library of Congress Control Number: 2007908863

ISBN 10: 0-9801469-0-9
ISBN 13: 978-0-9801469-0-5

*This book is dedicated to the people in our lives
who lift us, support us, and make us want
to become better people—our family.*

*My beautiful children Maximo and Veronica. It is because
of the love I have for you that I sat down one day, called Blanca
and decided to write this book. Thank you for your energy,
laughter, smiles, unconditional love and endless possibilities.*

*My friend, my love, my Michael.
Without you I couldn't have completed this book.
Thank you for your love and your patience. Always.*

*My sister, Diana, and my "brother" Mundi.
Even when I surprise you, which may be often, you
support me and believe in me. Thank you for your insight,
your wisdom, and your constant love. "Stay Gold."*

*My beautiful niece Ariel and nephews Alexander and
Andrew. You three came into my life before I had my own
children. You introduced me to a love I never had felt before.
Thank you for the light you shine upon us everyday.*

*Mami. Sin ti este libro nunca se hubiera completado.
Tu apollo y constante recordando me "porque yo no" es lo que una
madre ejemplar hace. Tu fortaleza me sorprende diariamente y
me hace querré ser mas como tu. I love you!*

*Papi. No estas aquí con nosotros físicamente pero se que el
empuje que sentí escribiendo este libro fue tuyo. Thank you for
always believing in me. The pride and love I saw everyday in
your eyes will remain with me forever. It is because of that love
and pride that I was able to believe in myself and complete this
book. You never let anyone stop you from doing what you
believed, one of the many things we have in common. I hope I
can continue your legacy and make you proud. I love you man!
Still my wind beneath my wings…thank you for helping me fly!*

Xoxoxo…Barbie

*To my running partner, friend and husband, Jeff.
Our first date was our first run, and nine years later
we're still at it. We ran six miles that day, and now we
still continue to maintain a great balance in our lives
that includes those six-miles-plus runs. Thank you for
being so supportive and understanding in our insane
and busy lives. If it weren't for you and your competitive
edge, I would never have had the courage to put my
workouts and thoughts into this book.*

*Alec and Jake…my twin boys. Wow! You are my life. Because
of you guys I found a love I thought I would never find. I never
imagined my life with twins, and now I can't imagine my life
without them. I love you both so much, and in years to come,
please, always know that Mami will always love you.*

*To my Mami and Papi. Gracias por el carino que seimpre nos
has dado. You have always been extremely supportive of whatever
I have chosen to do regardless of whether it was taking off to work
for Club Med or writing a book. Never doubting me, always
encouraging me. Because of that I am who I am today. I love you.*

My sister, Gisela. You have always inspired me to be everything I can. You are a very special person, and I want you to know that we all love you very much. You are real. You are true. Stay that way.

My brother, Henry. Thank you for being so supportive and believing in me in everything I do. And I have to also thank you, Luis. You have seen me in my insanity years when my brother was in Mexico and not there for me; you were his substitute. My brother always knew what to expect from me, but not you—you just went with it. To the both of you, I love you very much.

To Mimi and Pop-Pop. Thank you both for helping me out when I needed it the most. It means the world to me. Mimi, you are an amazing woman who is full of life and the desire to have fun, and I love that. And to you, Duke, just for being Duke.

To my sister-in-law, Donna, and my nephews, Zachary and Luke. Thank you for being so thoughtful and always thinking of us... Our lives sometimes get so busy, we forget those we shouldn't. I love you all and I want you never to forget that.

And to Barbie... Thank you for calling me like a madwoman and not asking me, but telling me we were writing a book! If it weren't for that seven a.m. phone call, I would never have done this.

Love, Blanca

Table of Contents

Acknowledgements

I could not have done this book without the help of my dear friend Blanca. Your endless energy inspires me and outlook on life motivates me. You pushed me when I doubted myself and my work. Our friendship has grown from kids playing with dolls to moms playing with kids. We share a common heartbreak but are able to take that negative experience and turn it into a positive one. We have learned what true friendship is about and luckily have found we have that with one another. Together we will help others in endless countless ways making a difference and setting the groundwork for those that follow.

We would like to acknowledge the following people with whom this book would have not been possible: Gilda Miqueli Jimenez, Mark Papianni, Christopher Toledo, Jennifer

Toledo, Alan Molina Esq., Maribel Quiala, Olga, Larry, Joel, Chris, Jessica and the team at Arbor Books. Regina, Carmela, Jean, and all my friends (big & small) at Marlboro Montessori Academy. And to the clients for their ongoing support throughout the years.

It is because of our firm belief in that everything does happen for a reason that we would like to also lastly acknowledge all those whom have touched our lives in good ways as well as bad. If it weren't for you we would not be here, in a very good place. So to all of you, thank you!

Introduction

Twenty years ago when I was seventeen, I picked up my first book on fitness and read it cover to cover in one day, and since then I have read just about every top seller fitness book known, and still continue to do so. My passion, which some may call an obsession, began early on in life with Jane Fonda workouts and early morning jogs with my sister and cousins when they would visit from New York. There was always some physical activity playing in my life whether it was dance classes, gymnastics, cheerleading or simply playing outside while bike riding with Blanca. It wasn't until recently that I took a deep look inside myself to try and figure out where this all stemmed from. I guess being a mom, I wanted to guard my children from all types of excessive behavior, and since at times the obsession of being thin was mine, I felt the need to figure out why.

I grew up in an amazing household of loving, caring, hard-working parents who arrived in this country as teenagers from Cuba. As exiles in a new country, life as many of you know was very difficult. My parents married and settled in New Jersey where there was a very big Cuban population. Our culture was never compromised, and, in fact, it was instilled in us in everything we did. We were Cuban-Americans and very proud of that. My multicultural Spanglish life began.

It wasn't until recently when my five-year-old son, who acted upon his male instinct to squeeze my ass, that it all came together. The men that I have been around since I was a kid—and still am—are fascinated by our biggest physical *asset*, our asses. As a child I remember "*que linda con su culo parado,*" and as a young girl entering her teen years the famous *piropos* began. Latin men (like most men) love our *assets*, and although it took me a long time to accept it, now I do, too.

So with that I ran to the phone, called Blanca and told her we were writing a book. I was going to share my experience of trying to achieve a body that was never going to be mine along with what has proven effective for me through years of research and studying the fascinating world of fitness. And she, who is considered an expert in her field, will provide us all with proven effective workouts to enhance the God blessed given curves and *caderas* we have as Latin woman. To wrap it up, since we love to eat and can never compromise our *comida criolla*, we have provided you with a few of our favorite dishes the healthy Latin way.

Con orgullo te presento the only guide to fitness you will ever need, *porque somos, y gracias a Dios que siempre seguiremos haciendo, Barbara por Atrás, Barbara por Alante, y Barbara por Adentro.* I hope you enjoy it!

Part 1
Nutrition

1
El Comienzo:
The Beginning

"…la vida es un carnaval, hay que vivir cantando…no hay que llorar…las penas se van cantando…" The song plays while I am running on my treadmill, sweating my butt off, at least trying to. But why? I came to the realization at that precise moment, while listening to the legendary Cuban artist Celia Cruz, that life is a carnival—a very fragile carnival that we must embrace and live, not waste away fighting a battle that will never be won. I will never look like those skinny models or friends for that matter because I, with pride and gratitude, am a Cuban-American woman who was blessed to be born with the asset of an ass. Yes, I have hips, thighs, and an ass. I enjoy *arroz con frijoles*, I love *tostones rellenos*, I melt over Cuban bread and savor every drop of a *cortadito. Soy Latina…Azucar!*

Blanca and I have been friends for as long as I can remember. We grew up a block away from one another in a small New Jersey town, where we both attended the same Catholic elementary school as well as the same public high school. Our passion and obsession with being fit began in the early nineties, crawling into the gym after a night of partying; sweating out the vodka and gin of the night before was our detox. Aerobics, weight training, spinning, group fitness, personal training, swimming, 'life guarding'—you name it, we did it and still do. After college I went on to work for a major automotive company. Married and two kids later, as was Blanca, I resigned and rejoined the fitness world that she had been mastering all along.

Seventeen years in the making! It took us many years of sweat and pain to get to this point, and we're still working on it. Yes, this is a lifestyle change and commitment for the long run. You will hear me saying this over and over throughout the book because I believe it is something we need to convince ourselves of and drill into our stubborn Latina heads. Everywhere we look there are quick fixes. Whether it's a pill to lose weight or a twenty-eight-day workout plan, they are out there. Did you ever stop and think why there is such a craze for email and texts? Everyone is on speed! We want quick results TODAY! Forget about emotional connections, "…click, click, click…next." So why should losing weight and working towards achieving a healthy lifestyle be any different? We want to lose weight fast for that wedding, party, or vacation. It seems that once we reach our goals, out come the *pastelitos* or cookies and we are back where we started. This viscous cycle continues over and over, and we find ourselves spending our precious lives on a "diet," frustrated because we are out of shape. Ladies, we need to stop this madness! Yes, it's going to be hard because we need a large amount of patience, something many of us lack. We feel as though the world is working against us in overdrive, but if we could at least start with one thing we could slowly work on the others. So let's begin with fitness.

After the birth of my third child I felt lost. I have always been the type of person to enjoy dressing and looking good. I abandoned that person but found her again when I met Barbara and started training with her. Her outlook on life gave me the push I needed, and her love for food taught me that I can still enjoy the things I love without losing who I am. Today I am a better person and above all a better mother. Thank you!

—Christina

2

"Santa Barbara... santa por alante y barbara por atras..."

Pues aquí vamos. Can you hear them saying it? I sure can; "*que rica estas*"..."*estas por la maseta*"..."*que nalgas mas buena tienes*"..."*si cocina como caminas me como hasta la raspa...*"

I grew up hearing these famous *piropos* as I would walk to the corner bodega running errands for my mom or dad. It may be crazy, but after a while I kind of liked it. I felt as if they were something of an ego boost. Yes I have an ass, and I like it! Gracias! We have curves. We are voluptuous. We have hips that don't lie, and oh, are we going to use them!

Who out there listens to her body? I mean really listens? Wouldn't you pay attention to an unusual clatter in your car? Or how about an irregular sound or smell in your home? Listening to your body is one of the most important things you need to do in order to keep your health intact. I can tell you exactly when I am ovulating or precisely what will happen to my body if I eat a *natilla con dulce leche*. Have you ever tried this most incredible dessert? Amazing! There is a spot in Miami called *Molinas* that serves it just right. Try it and you will remember me. Following your first taste, for one is all you can have (this is a fitness book, remember), you can do what a dear friend of mine did the first time we went. Simply rub your spoon on the floor and you will no longer be tempted to eat it! Next, you must make sure the server takes it away before you grab someone else's spoon, which is certainly something I would do. Being capable of doing so requires willpower, determination, and honesty. The bottom line is we all want and need to be happy. So, if fitness and being healthy is your thing, then let's work together. It doesn't matter who you are; all people should join in, but we Latinas have certain areas we need to focus on, which is why we will share our experience and success with you. *Para sequir la tradicion y orgullo de tener un tremendo cuerpo!*

Growing up, I heard all the sayings, and perhaps it is why I felt the need to melt my body away with every diet out there. I can honestly say I've been on a diet practically my whole life—well, except during my two pregnancies when I gained over seventy pounds each one because I ate everything in sight. I've tried them all: three-day diets, grapefruit diets,

Atkins diet, Jenny Craig; you name it, I've tried it. Of course, every time I started a new diet program I lost weight and thought, "How wonderful, this one is it! It really works! I am losing weight!" It wasn't until the birth of my first-born when I realized all these diets worked because I was shocking my system and introducing it to something new. This is why you automatically lose weight when starting something new, whether it's an exercise program or diet. After a while of doing the same exercise routine or food regiment, your body gets used to it and you no longer lose weight or see the results. Change is important in every aspect of life. Not only will *you* get bored, but your body will as well. This is why it is crucial for you to add variety within your exercise routine and meals. In the chapters ahead we will talk about eating in moderation and portion control. We will explain "cheat treat days" and how they could ultimately work for you. Some people don't believe in that one day to cheat and eat those foods they have so diligently stayed away from, as they fear they will not be able to fully stop the eating and once again regain self control. I unfortunately was one of those people. Through my own experiences I have learned eating in moderation works best within my lifestyle. I love chocolate, bread and wine, and if you told me that I could no longer enjoy these, especially after the crazy lifestyles we women lead, *te mandaria para el carajo.* Upon realizing that completely excluding these treats from my daily diet would surely lead to my insanity, I opted for portion control and creative cooking, and most importantly heavy-duty exercise. Yes, ladies, it's common science; eat less, exercise more. How many times have we heard "you are what you eat?" Unfortunately, it is true! If you want to eat *masita de puerco con arroz y platanos maduros* everyday, you will become a fried pig!

Growing up in a Latin household was not easy on many levels. In addition to having chaperons and your occasional *chancleta* thrown at you, we did not eat very well either. Looking back, there are a number of things I would change, but I realize my parents did the best that they could with the information they had at the time. Unfortunately for my parents, it took me thirty-seven years to realize how much they did for me and what a challenge parenting is. So *mami, y papi donde estes, gracias otra vez.*

Now, let's get back to food. While growing up, focusing on eating healthy food was not a top priority. My parents were fantastic cooks, and they really knew how to accent the flavors of true Latin cooking. It was traditional for family members to pass along compliments saying I looked good, but good in our family meant that I was twenty pounds over-weight.

It is no secret that we Latinos as a culture love meat; as it is the men love a good amount of meat on their plates as well as on their women! Unfortunately for us Latinas we will do anything we can to avoid the meat which sticks to our thighs and seems almost impossible to eliminate. Since a meat diet is custom in our culture, we have learned to live with it and finally embrace it. In later chapters I've provided many recipes that allow you to enjoy healthy meals while not abandoning your craving for meat!

"La dieta se empieza mañana" o "eso no engorda, un día no hace nada." How many times have we prolonged starting the diet just one more day? So instead, let's eat today and starve ourselves tomorrow. It's unfortunate that when someone says "diet," you automatically have a negative feeling about it. "Oh, I have to go on a diet," or "I'll start my diet in the morning," or even worse, "On New Year's Day I will begin my diet." Do we not realize that a diet is everything we eat on a daily basis, both good and bad? So, why is it that we have come to associate the word diet solely with healthy foods? A diet could also be junk food. Let's start by removing diet from our vocabulary since it's only going to set us up for failure. "Healthy lifestyle," now that's a better phrase—daily choices we make to be healthy while not losing who we are. Ultimately, our main goal in life is being happy and at peace with ourselves. That sounds much better and it already gives you a sense of acceptance, a promising and positive outlook on your new, healthy life plan.

When I decided I needed help to get into the best shape I could for my son's wedding, I naturally turned to Blanca for help. I had taken her spin classes and enjoyed her motivation and determination to push everyone to their limits. I thought it would be a short term solution but more than 5 years later I continue to be trained by her. At 50 I feel and look much younger than I did 10 years ago and I owe it all to Blanca.

—Maritza

3
Todo lo Exagerado es Malo

Pero lo somo. Somo exajerago de naturaleza. We love to look hot. We love our stilettos. We love to be loud. We love to stand out! So, because this is our nature we will both jump into this full force and dig deep within ourselves to make the commitment in changing our lifestyle.

Feeling nostalgic for a place I called home for six years, I was drawn to Dr. Agatston's *South Beach Diet*. Its concept is one that I still follow today; however, the way I initially approached it was completely wrong. The *South Beach Diet* explains the importance of removing the "bad carbohydrates" from our diets—what I and many call the "white stuff." As a Latin woman this *could* be very difficult. I still remember the look on my father's face the day I told him I was never going to eat white rice or white bread again. Unfortunately, that day is connected to the last few days I spent with him. He died of a massive heart attack three days later over Thanksgiving weekend. Although my father ate well, genetics won the battle. Heart disease runs in my family, which provides much motivation in my mission to live and practice a healthy lifestyle.

Minimizing the "white stuff" such as white rice, yellow rice, and white bread as well as altering your life through the inclusion of whole grains will help you feel and look better, while adding years to your life. I am not saying never to eat those items again, but to slightly alter what you have been used to. And, to make it even easier, everyone is jumping on the wagon. Not long ago, while shopping at my local market I was very happy to see that GOYA even has *arroz integral* now. Brown rice is delicious and a plate of it with black beans is an amazingly healthy dish. But it is crucial you stop there! *El bistecito* has to be kept for another meal. Later on you will see how I have put together some of my favorite dishes so you, too, could enjoy the healthy Latina way!

Let's take a quick look at how carbs work because as we all know, rice and tortillas are a big part of our diet and both are considered a "bad carb" to so many nutritionists out there. All carbs contain sugars which exist in many different forms, from simple table sugar to fructose which is found in fruit. The more sugar a food has, such as a candy bar, the faster it is released into your blood system, known to many as the "sugar rush." Our bodies treat all carbs basically the same way; we digest the food we have eaten and either burn or store the fuel produced by the carbs. The problem arises when we begin to store more fuel then we burn, turning it into body fat. Combining and adding different healthy foods to your diet will slow down the sugar process and be an asset in burning fat.

Fiber is one of those marvelous healthy additions that will slow down sugar. Adding fiber to your carbs such as grains will make your stomach work harder, slow down digestion, and avoid any quick entry of sugar into your bloodstream. There will be no quick sugar rushes or drops, and you will remain satisfied for a longer period of time. If you are going to eat carbs it is important that you slow down the digestive process. Extra virgin olive oil (EVOO), tomatoes, spinach, and broccoli are all great supplements which you can add to your carbs to make them a healthier alternative while slowing down the blood sugar release in your system. For example, we love rice, but alone it is not the healthiest choice of carbohydrate from a nutritionist's perspective. When prepared with other ingredients, such as beans, you have successfully turned a grain that is considered "unacceptable" into a very healthy meal which will help you achieve your goal of health and lifelong fitness.

Take a look at the top power foods: olive oil, grapes, tomatoes, peppers, almonds, and berries, to name a few. They come from the Mediterranean, and yes, many of us Latinos come from Spain. So why is it we have neglected to add these nutrient enriched foods into our daily lifestyle? A lot of us eat simply because we are hungry, but if we would instead think of it as an art of tasting, rather than eating to live, the battle would be half won. We Latinos love to get together with family; granted we all know each other and *everyone* is family, therefore we tend to have large gatherings. The joy of eating, drinking, and talking is endless, and for us Cubans our *"cuando yo vivia en Cuba"* stories are historic. How amazing is it going to be when you no longer feel guilty the next day for having that *Mojito* with *tapas*, and know that you and your body enjoyed a wonderful time, *y que se repite*!

Now that we are done talking lets get down to business. Stand up, raise your hands, and repeat after me (yes the cheerleader in me is coming out)…

"Tenemos Caderas"
"Tenemos Murlos"
"Tenemos Nalagas"
"Tenemos Curvas"
"Tenemos Tetas"
"Tenemos Sangre"

"Somos Latinas!!!"
"AZUCAR!!!!!!!"

Blanca has been essential in my weight loss. She has taught me how to exercise, and pushed me beyond my comfort zone. Now, I actually enjoy it! I lost 65 pounds and have kept it off for over a year! I owe it all to Blanca.
—Jennifer

4

A Comer...

When looking to achieve a balanced life of healthy food and exercise you must look deep inside yourself as well as your kitchen and ask, "Am I ready to do this?" If the answer is no, please read no further and close the book. I am sure there is a quick fix pill out there for you. If you said yes, then let's get moving!

I believe being organized in life is the key to success in anything you do. That being said, your kitchen is certainly not the exception. When planning your meals, think a week in advance; give yourself an idea of what it is you want to cook for the week and shop accordingly. It is so important that you train your body and your mind on your healthy eating habits. Deprivation is the key to failure; therefore it is important that you allow yourself to eat every two to three hours. You will have your three main meals with two snacks in between. Breakfast, lunch and dinner with a mid-morning and mid-afternoon snack. This way you are always satisfied and are also training your metabolism to continuously burn excess calories and fat. Planning your shopping list accordingly will avoid binge eating, ordering takeout, and quick non-healthy meal alternatives. Start writing your shopping list whichever day you begin your week, whether it's Saturday, Sunday, or Monday with those ingredients you may need. I prefer to organize myself with a mental diagram of the market I am going to. For example, my favorite super-market starts with the produce department, then fruits, breads, bakery, and ends with dairy. Based on the layout I complete my shopping list in that order, making it easier for me to stick to what I need, avoiding temptation at all levels.

Ever since I can remember, in school we learned about the importance of nutrition and the food groups in the 'Food Guide Pyramid' as set by the U.S. Department of Agriculture. Everything is explained and written out for us: the amount of servings we should eat from the grains, vegetables, fruits, proteins, and dairy groups, in addition to sparingly using fats, oils, and sweets. Did we ever follow these recommendations at home? I am sorry, but green beans and carrots were not our thing growing up. We had white rice with every meal, and if I were to tell my mother today to eliminate her rice she would look me in the eyes, 'yes, dear,' me, and continue on her *arroz* merry way. *Arroz con frijoles, arroz con huevo frito, arroz con sardinas, arroz con gandules, arroz con salchichas, arroz con vegetales, arroz con leche! Arroz, arroz, arroz…* Our parents and ancestors ate rice, *arepas*, and any other "unacceptable" grains daily and stayed fit for one reason and one reason alone: they worked out without even realizing it. They walked everywhere and used their natural physical strength to do everything from carpentry to laundry. Today, in our country we have everything at our fingertips. We don't have to get out of bed or off the couch to turn on the TV, and we are ever so intrigued and delighted to hear that there are other technological advances in the making that will actually do even more for us! Yippee!! So it's no wonder why we are overweight and out of shape.

There are an increasing number of Hispanic Americans in our country with diabetes. Out of the thirty million people approximately two million have been diagnosed with diabetes. On an average we are one point nine times more likely to have diabetes than non-Hispanic whites. It is twice as common in those of Mexican American and Puerto Rican descent and although lower in Cuban-Americans, it is still higher than among the non-Hispanic whites. Most Hispanic Americans with diabetes have type two which could be treated with diet and exercise. Specifically designed for those with diabetes and health practitioners like myself who want to make our Latino brothers and sisters healthier, the traditional food pyramid has just gotten a Latin makeover. A *new* food pyramid has been introduced by the Latino Nutrition Coalition, The Traditional Healthy Latin American Diet Pyramid. Take a look at their website, www.latinonnutrition.org. Not only is the website informative, but it also provides great Latino recipes geared towards improving our health. The Latin American Diet Pyramid is based on the U.S. Department of Agriculture, with an emphasis on the favorite foods we eat such as pork, tortillas, rice, beans, yuca, mangos, avocados, and chilies. The Latin American Diet Pyramid is broken down into basically three parts: What to consume at every meal, daily, and weekly—1) Fruits, grains, and vegetables should be eaten at every meal, 2) Dairy, poultry, and fish should be eaten daily, 3) Limit the meat and sweets to once a week, which could be consumed on your "treat cheat day."

Later on we will talk about portion control and visualizing your meals by balancing them. The amount of foods from each group is very important in maintaining a healthy lifestyle; however, it is equally important to keep track as to the time of day you are eating them. It is very important that you begin your days eating your grains and carbs. Throughout the day slowly minimize your carb intake and

Latin American Diet Pyramid

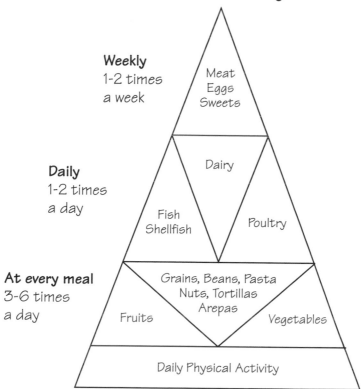

Weekly
1-2 times
a week

Meat
Eggs
Sweets

Daily
1-2 times
a day

Dairy

Fish
Shellfish

Poultry

At every meal
3-6 times
a day

Grains, Beans, Pasta
Nuts, Tortillas
Arepas

Fruits

Vegetables

Daily Physical Activity

stick to your vegetables and protein. Your snacks could be anything from a piece of fruit, a light yogurt, or a few almonds with cottage cheese and blueberries; whatever you choose make sure you stay on track with your new lifestyle. Also, avoid at all costs eating a big meal for dinner followed by lounging on your couch with your favorite *novela*. If your schedule doesn't accommodate an early meal, it is essential to go for a walk or engage in some type of exercise to burn off those calories. I like to have my last bite of whatever at least two hours before going to bed, so it is important for me to choose a meal with significant nutritional value. Our relatives across the pond have the right idea; when studying abroad in Spain I was very interested in learning of how the locals had dinner so late at night. Little did I realize that their biggest meal was at lunch time, "la comida," and their dinner, "la cena," consisted of a very light meal, wine and plenty of conversation. Some may say that is unrealistic for us over here with our conflicting schedules; however, I am sure that if you really put your mind to it you can figure out a way to make it work for you as well.

It is crucial for us all to carry healthy options in our kitchen. We all have different tastes, but one trait we have in common is that we want to be healthy. How can we not be concerned with taking care of the most precious gift that has been given to us, our bodies? Think back to the best gift you have ever received, whether it was as a child or an adult. Possibly, it was your favorite doll or bike or car; regardless of what it was, ask yourself one thing: did you take care of it? Do you still?? Why is it that so many of us treat the most precious gift our creator has given us so poorly? How ungrateful are we? How do you feel when you put all your heart and soul into a project or gift and the receiver just brushes it off and doesn't care about it? Let's think of our bodies as this amazing gift that must be nourished and cherished to honor ourselves and the person who brought us here.

Our personal touches in the kitchen and the dishes we prepare will be the key to staying on track with healthy food and meal choices. Understanding how your body works and why you should put certain foods into it over others will help you in your cooking, eating and staying fit. The satisfaction of achieving your fitness goals will make you feel as you did when you finally understood how to solve that math problem that was driving you crazy all semester! Along with your newfound confidence you'll feel the power to make your own right choices. Being creative and trying new and different dishes as you go along will give you a result you'll be proud of, and not to mention those enjoying your concoctions will have something to rave about!!

I've been working out since 1997 when I was twenty-one. It wasn't until April in 2005 that I decided to seek the help of a certified personal trainer. I was extremely fortunate to have met Blanca and owe to her the huge difference I feel and see in my body today. Not only has my body mass index decreased, but I have become leaner and above all have been able to maintain the weight and change. Education on fitness and nutrition is very important to me, and luckily I have been able to learn both from her. Thank you!

—Paula

5
Nutrition Facts

Before we go grocery shopping it is important that we all know how to read a nutrition label; therefore, I am going to give you a brief explanation of one.

Serving Size: The amount of food, as explained, which is used to determine the nutritional facts.

Servings Per Container: The amount of servings the package contains.

Calories and Calories from Fat: The amount of calories in the serving in addition to the amount you are getting from fat. There are good fats out there such as EVOO, so don't let this number scare you if it is high. Typically, you should try to take in no more than two thousand calories on a daily basis.

Total Fat: Adds the fat grams from all types of fat: saturated, trans, polyunsaturated, and monounsaturated. Saturated fats generally can be found in red meats and red meat products, such as lamb, beef, pork, and even some dairy products. Poly and mono can typically be found in plant oils such as olive, canola, peanut, safflower, sunflower, corn, or soybean oils. Unfortunately, trans-fats can be associated with the goodies (cookies, crackers, and cakes). Poly and mono are the good fats here. I like to stay away from the other two and typically keep the intake of them to a bare minimum.

Cholesterol: The total milligrams of cholesterol. Another item that should be limited. The American Heart Association recommends consuming less than three hundred milligrams per day, while the average daily intake for men is three hundred sixty and two hundred forty for women.

Sodium: The total milligrams of sodium per serving. Another count that I like to keep at a minimum, especially with high blood pressure and cholesterol issues in my family. The average is twenty-three hundred milligrams per day, though this number can fluctuate depending on the types of food you consume. Although twenty-three hundred seems like a high number, a single teaspoon of salt can provide a day's worth of sodium! This being said, if you are looking to minimize your daily intake of sodium, it is wise to avoid eating foods containing salt.

Total Carbohydrates: The total grams of every type of carb. As we discussed earlier, carbohydrates act as fuel for your body as does gasoline for your vehicle. Depending on your diet, a common intake of carbs ranges from about two hundred to three hundred grams.

Dietary Fiber: The total grams of fiber in each serving. I like to make sure I have at least three grams of fiber in each serving. When planning your meals, it is important to have between twenty to twenty-five grams on a daily basis, for increasing fiber within your meal plan will promote normal elimination of waste products of digestion.

Sugar: The amount of sugar in each serving. There is no minimum of sugar one should be consuming daily, though it is recommended that we do not exceed fifty grams. For the calorie counters out there, sugar is not the way to go, for it contains calories but nothing else.

Protein: The total grams of protein in each serving. Daily recommendations show a minimum of at least fifty grams, which can easily be accomplished. Proteins are abundant in eggs, chicken, beef, and peanut butter, to name a few. An important factor to be aware of is along with protein comes cholesterol, fat, and carbohydrates, so it is important to monitor your intake.

Vitamins and Minerals: It is required that all food labels have the recommended daily values as opposed to the grams or milligrams in each serving. A great source of your daily vitamins and minerals can be obtained through fruits and vegetables, as well as multivitamins.

Ingredients: The list of food ingredients listed in order based on their weight.

Shopping list: Here are some of my favorites...

Vegetables

Vegetables, whether they are frozen, fresh, or canned are a great source of vitamins and nutrients. The one drawback of fresh vegetables is that they must be eaten in a given period of time, as opposed to canned and frozen which never spoil. Most vegetables will remain fresh for a period of at least a week and sometimes longer when they are properly kept. Canned fruits and vegetables are often considered nutritionally inferior to their fresh and frozen counterparts. This is true when it comes to salt and sugar content, and as we discussed above, in the type of lifestyle we are hoping to achieve, we want to minimize their intake. The main asset in buying canned fruits and vegetables is they are usually processed immediately following harvest, which is when their nutrient content is at its peak.

Regardless of how you buy your fruits and vegetables, it is essential you incorporate them into your daily eating regiment, as per the Latin American Diet Pyramid. Below you can find a list of my favorite vegetables which provide the daily nutrients essential to living a healthy lifestyle.

Asparagus	Cabbage
Beans, *all*	Carrots
Bell Peppers, *all colors*	Cauliflower
Broccoli	Celery

Chili Pepper

Corn

Cucumber

Eggplant

Green Onion

Spinach

Lettuce, *all kinds*

(I love the ready bags!)

Squash

Sweet Potato

Tomato

Zucchini

Avocado w/tomatoes and red onion, drizzle with EVOO, salt and pepper, and basil on wheat or pumpernickel bagel...riquisimo!

Fruits

It's no secret I am a big fan of fruit, for it is a quick and easy way to get your daily portion of vitamins and nutrients.!!! Fruits are fresh and light and good with just about anything! From cereal to salads, cocktails to *congris*, adding fruit is the way to a healthier and hotter Latina! There are *thousands* of different types of fruit out there, all of which provide us with strong health benefits. It's recommended we eat at least five pieces of fruit daily to achieve maximum health benefits, and below is a brief list to help you reach that number.

Apples

Avocado

Bananas

Berries of all kinds

Grapefruit

Kiwi

Lemon

Lime

Mangoes	Peaches
Melons, *all kinds*	Pears
Oranges	Pineapple
Papaya	Plums

Mango salsa on everything and anything...mango cut in chunks, one half a red onion chopped, two tbsp lime juice, dash salt & pepper, and tbsp cilantro. Mix, chill, and serve!

Protein

Below is a list of high protein foods, along with the amount of protein per serving. Following this guide will help you plan your meals accordingly to ensure you're getting sufficient daily amounts.

Egg Whites or Substitute—one large egg contains six grams of protein.

Beans, garbanzos, black, red kidney, lentil, split peas—one half cup of cooked beans contains between seven to ten grams of protein.

Beef, all lean cuts—most cuts of beef contain seven grams of protein per ounce of meat. *Sirloin, Tenderloin, Top round*

Dairy
  Milk, fat free/two
      percent—one cup
      contains eight grams
      of protein.
  Yogurt, light/fat-free/
      low-fat—one cup
      usually contains
      between eight to
      twelve grams, depend-
      ing on brand.
  Cheese, low-fat
      Soft cheeses
      (Mozzarella, Brie,
      Camembert)—
      six grams of protein
      per ounce.
      Medium cheeses
      (Cheddar, Swiss)—
      seven or eight
      grams per ounce.
      Hard cheeses
      (Parmesan)—ten
      grams per ounce.

Fish, all kinds—most fish
    contain six grams per
    ounce; a six-ounce
    can of tuna contains
    forty grams.

Pork, all lean cuts
Tenderloin—four ounces
    contains twenty-nine
    grams
Boiled Ham—three ounces
    contains nineteen grams
Ground pork—three ounces
    cooked contains
    twenty-two grams
Bacon—one slice contains
    three grams
Canadian-style Bacon—
    one slice contains
    five to six grams

Poultry, white meat no skin
Chicken Breast—three and
    one half ounces contains
    thirty grams

Turkey Breast—three
   ounces contains
   twenty-five grams
Turkey Bacon—one piece
   contains two grams

Shellfish, all kinds
Lobster—three and one half
   ounces contains
   twenty-one grams
Crab—three ounces
   contains nineteen grams
Shrimp—four ounces
   (about ten shrimp)
   contains eighteen grams

*One half cup cottage cheese w/blueberries and almonds...
perfectly nutritious snack!*

Nuts

The following information is based on three and one half ounces:

Peanut butter, low fat or all
   natural—contains
   twenty-two grams
Peanuts—contain
   twenty-five grams

Almonds—contain
   twenty-one grams
Cashews—contain
   twenty grams

Grains
At least three percent dietary fiber

Bread	Cereal
Multigrain, Oat & Bran, Rye, Pumpernickel, Whole Wheat	Oatmeal *(not instant)*, Fiber One, All Bran
	Pasta
	Wheat, Brown Rice, Tortillas

Pan con mantequilla…use light butter.
Smart Balance is…delicioso!

Condiments

Extra Virgin Olive Oil *(EVOO)*	Goya Adobo
	Dry White Cooking Wine
Vinegar	Red Cooking Wine
Pam	Smart Balance Light Butter
Low-fat Mayo	Salsa
Mustard	Sugar Substitute

And every spice out there that does not contain sugar

Snacks

Low sugar/sugar free snacks

Ice cream	Gelatin
Ice pops	Pudding
Fudge pops	Semi-Sweet chocolate
Galletas Maria	Dark chocolate
Gum	Whipped Cream

Beverages

Water, *all kinds*	Juice
Coffee	Soda
Tea	Wine, Red/White
Sugar-free drinks	

Café con Leche…try two percent or skim steamed or heated in a saucepan w/splenda & cinnamon…un amor

6
Portion Control

I like following the visual plan when I serve and eat my meals. By being able to envision the dish as I prepare it, I ensure myself that I am able to include food from all of the necessary groups to achieve optimum nutrition.

Breakfast

It's always been said that breakfast is the most important meal of the day. Regardless of whether or not you prefer your breakfast in a dish or a bowl, I have devised a system to help ensure adequate portioning of the daily essentials. For example, rather than solely consuming an entire egg white omelet, go ahead and only make half of what you usually would. My personal favorite addition which spices up any omelet is vegetable and salsa. Such a minor addition not only adds a lot of flavor to an ordinary egg white omelet, but it also takes care of your vegetable serving.

Now to top off the meal toast yourself up a piece of whole wheat bread (lightly butter it if you prefer), and serve it along with a small portion of berries or any other fruit. And of course a cold glass of skim or low-fat milk complements any meal! Not only do you have a delicious meal at your fingertips, but by dividing each food group into small portions you make sure you cover all the groups in the Latino Food Pyramid. If you don't have the time to make a breakfast as discussed above, serve yourself one half a cup of cereal such as *Fiber One* with a cup of skim or low-fat milk. Always finish off your breakfast with a piece of fruit. It's healthy, filled with great carbs and nutrients and a fabulous way to start your day.

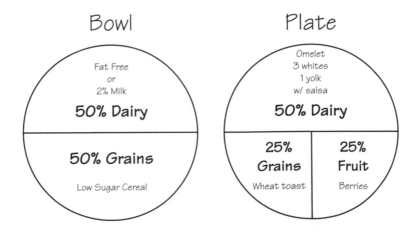

Bowl

Fat Free
or
2% Milk

50% Dairy

50% Grains

Low Sugar Cereal

Plate

Omelet
3 whites
1 yolk
w/ salsa

50% Dairy

**25%
Grains**

**25%
Fruit**

Wheat toast

Berries

Your mid-morning and mid-afternoon snack should be something light and healthy. I noted a few earlier; however a few of my favorites are low fat cheese or a small apple with peanut butter. Whatever you may choose keep it small and satisfying so that you are not rabid when its time for lunch!

Lunch and Dinner

When it comes to lunch and dinner, you can eat similar meals as long as you are eating the right foods. Remember, as stated in an earlier chapter, you want to eat the majority of your carbs in the daytime so you have time to burn them off. Since we're trying to gradually minimize the intake of grains later in the day, focus on filling up with the other food groups; that way you will be full and won't be tempted to indulge in carbs late at night. I can't express enough how unused carbs simply turn to fat!

To ensure that I cover all of the food groups in either my lunch or my dinner, I like to follow equal portions such as twenty-five percent of each group across the board.

Balance out your dish with equal amounts of protein, grains, vegetables, and fruit. *Todo con moderación no solo en la comida pero en todos aspectos de la vida.* It's crucial to success in all you do!

When you have reached your target weight, it is okay to indulge and treat yourself to a "cheat" day. This will be one

Lunch and Dinner

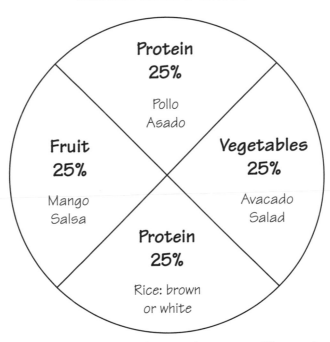

day in the week of your choice when you will eat whatever you like. That wasn't a misprint; *yes, whatever you like!* Shocking isn't it, but so true! Not only will you enjoy those foods you have been missing, but you will also be shocking your system. Once you return to your normal *new* eating habits your body will continue to lose weight and burn fat and calories. You have worked very hard and deserve your indulgence. It is important to never deprive yourself of the things you enjoy because like so many of us you will binge and make yourself sick. I cannot begin to tell you how many times in my life I have done just that. And as you are reading and probably shaking your head in agreement I know so many other ladies out there who are with me on this one. It's sick but true! Binge eating affects three point five percent of women. We get so crazed in the 'must lose weight fast life' that we deprive ourselves of the things we love, leaving us to at any given moment lose control and attack the kitchen, in turn making ourselves sick physically and mentally. So this is why I stress that it is so important that we moderate our food intake and never leave out something we love. It is best that you give yourself one "treat cheat day," but if you have binge eating tendencies and don't think you can make it to that one day, then allow yourself one small piece of your favorite "treat" when you get the craving. In order to practice moderation you must be honest and true to yourself. Remember, one day a week of cheating is okay, but if you begin to notice it becoming a once-a-day occurrence, you must rat yourself out and seek the discipline that got you this far! Keep in mind there is nothing better than the feeling of accomplishment. We praise our children from the moment they enter our worlds with phrases such as "good jobs" and "way to go." Our bosses or partners in life share in our ego boosts as well, promoting us and praising us with affirmations when we succeed. So, just imagine how fantastic a feeling it will be when you've made it the whole week or day without having that guilty pleasure! Remember, pleasure is an amazing feeling that will only give you added positive results in everything you do, but guilt will only spiral into more of the negatives. So let's just stay away from those "guilty pleasures" and stick to long lasting,

"I did it!" positive pleasures!!

Part 2
The Workout

7

Before You Start

Although eating right is extremely important to achieving a healthier lifestyle, working out is the piece of the puzzle that cannot be left out. Both are equal in value and need to be approached with the same discipline and frame of mind. You must maintain a positive outlook to embrace and accept the new lifestyle and lifelong commitment.

The following workout has been proven effective by many of Blanca's clients throughout the years, as you have read throughout the book within the testimonials. Some exercises have been altered and mastered to meet current standards. In addition, she has chosen certain exercises that will be aimed with an added focus on our Latin assets. The core areas will be the buttocks (of course), thighs, abs, arms and back.

So, before you start your workout routine close your eyes and envision yourself dancing along to salsa, merengue, or to the dance of your choice shaking your beautiful Latin hips. *Porque gracias a Dios lo tenemos, la sangre y el amor de ser Latina!*

¡Adelante!

When I was looking for a personal trainer I wanted someone who was Latin and new the struggles we as Latinas have with our assets and eating habits. I was thrilled when I was referred to Blanca. Today I owe my body, self-esteem, and new outlook on life to her!

—Laura

8
Ready to Sweat!
La Tortura

There is nothing like a good sweat when working out. If done correctly you will sweat like you never have and enjoy doing so, while seeing results! Don't ever say you can't do it, because then you won't. Once you incorporate the word 'can't' into your vocabulary you are setting yourself up for failure. Constantly tell yourself you *can* and you ultimately *will.* This is going to be a challenge. Life is about challenges; without them our lives wouldn't be complete.

Please be advised that it is important that you consult a physician before beginning this or any new exercise program.

Here we go...we will be introducing you to two different workouts. The first is for those who have worked out before, while the second is meant for those who have not. Upon determining which category you fall into, whether you are a beginner, intermediate, or advanced, the next step is to obtain a few necessary pieces of equipment. For the workouts we will be discussing, you will need a stability ball and weights. I recommend three pounds for the beginner, five pounds for the intermediate and ten pounds for those who feel they are advanced. However, you will be using two different sets of weights— one for the category you are currently in, and one for the next level up. For example, if you are a beginner you will start using the three pound weights and finish with the five pound. Throughout the workout you will be doing two sets of fifteen reps for each exercise. A rep can be defined as one completed movement. It is crucial to always keep your body fully engaged at all times, bellies and butts tight. Even if you are not working on a particular area, keeping the other muscle groups tight and engaged will activate their energy and work their magic. This is an intense workout with little room for breaks. You will be moving constantly. Sips of water are allowed, but no minute breaks. We want you to keep your heart rate elevated and continue burning fat throughout the routine. We will be incorporating what is called compound exercises. These are moves that involve more than one joint, such as squats and lunges, which activate more total muscle increasing calorie burn and strength. The more muscles you work, the more calories will be burned. Working out with free weights force you to use other muscles in your body through alignments, form, and stability, as you are engaging your whole body.

Now let's get to work! *A comenzar la tortura!*

Workout will take twenty-five to thirty minutes to complete.

This workout should be done 3-4 times a week for optimal results with either a rest day in-between or walk exercise day 3, 4, or 5. For the ultimate challenge implement walk exercise day 6 or 7. Totaling a 5-6 day workout week. As with this or any workout routine, although you want to take your muscles to the point of fatigue (feel the soreness) it is very important that you listen to your body and not take it beyond its limits. You will reach your target weight and fitness goal, *no te desesperes,* patience is key to everything in life.

Figures 1 and 2

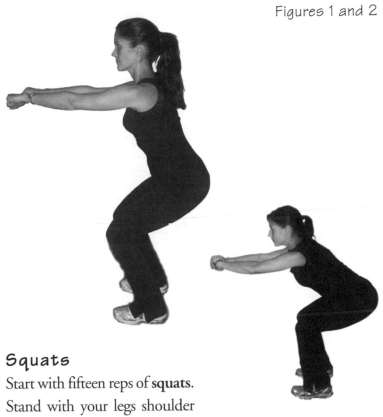

Squats

Start with fifteen reps of **squats**.
Stand with your legs shoulder
width apart. Bend the legs at knees lowering your torso
between your legs never letting your knees pass your toes.
Bring yourself back up again in standing position and repeat.

After the fifteenth rep stay in squat position and hold it
for ten seconds, intermediate and advanced follow up with
jump squats for fifteen reps (Beginners skip the jump squats
and go to next exercise). See fig. 1 and 2.

Figures 3 and 4

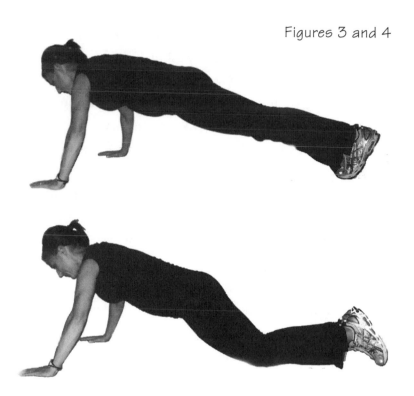

Pushups

Following the completion of the fifteenth rep of your jump squats, immediately get into **pushup** position for fifteen reps; for those beginners start on your knees, and the more advanced begin with legs extended following a full range of motion. See fig. 3 and 4.

Dips

Upon completion of your set of pushups, quickly get back up to squat position and repeat the first set of squats, jump squats (advanced and intermediate only) and pushups.

Dips are a great 'at home workout,' for they target muscles in both the **triceps** as well as the chest. All you need is any kind of chair, and you are ready to begin!

- Start by putting the back of the chair against a wall.
- Place your hands firmly on the edge of the seat, so that your knuckles are pointing forward.
- Place your legs out in front of you, in a ninety degree angle, while making sure your feet are pointing forward with your toes up.
- Make sure your shoulders stay down and back, and that your elbows stay tightly against your sides.
- Slowly bend your elbows down into a ninety degree angle and pause, then return to the original position, putting pressure on the heels of your hands.

Through this exercise you will feel a burn in the back of your arms, don't be alarmed, as this means you are properly executing the exercise.

For a beginner, the stability ball may appear overwhelming at first glance. But don't be turned away, for the ball is ideal for improving functional strength, flexibility, and balance.

Maintaining proper alignment on the stability ball energizes the body's natural reflexes and encourages the body to react as a completely integrated unit. Each movement challenges the entire body to work together in order to maintain correct posture and balance. Perform the following motions resting less than a minute in between each set.

Position yourself on the stability ball and grab your weights. Sit upright on the ball with your arms and elbows bent so that the dumbbell is behind your head; the movement consists of straightening your arms as you press the weights toward the

Figure 6

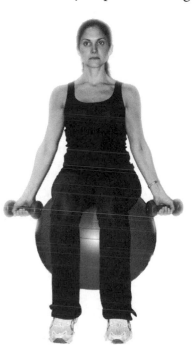

ceiling. It is normal to feel a burning sensation in your **triceps** as it is a sign of doing the exercise correctly!

Perform fifteen reps, and upon completion of the last rep, go back to dips for 15 reps followed by behind your head tricep extensions.

Position yourself back on the stability ball grab light weight (a lot of reps involved so do go light) and place them on your sides with hand facing forward *see fig.6 bring weights up in a curl motion at your shoulder level turn your palms to face out and perform over head press *see fig. 7 & 8. Do 15 reps. After your 15th rep stay in the over head press position and do 15 more reps of just **shoulder presses** (this is totally going to bring your shoulder muscles to the point of fatigue , don't give up just get thru it). Once you have completed 15 straight over-head presses stay in shoulder press position and perform counts of two up two down presses (instead of going up all the way you stop mid way, hold, and then go up to final position and back down for the two count again) This is called up 2 down 2…do 10 reps.

Upon completion of the two up, two down set of ten, complete one final set of fifteen shoulder presses and then put the weights down.

Figures 7 and 8

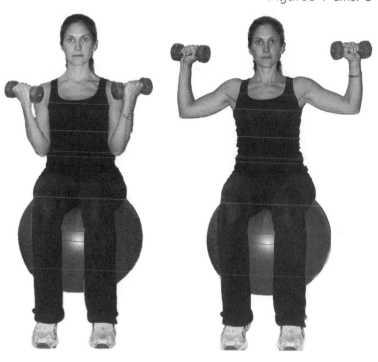

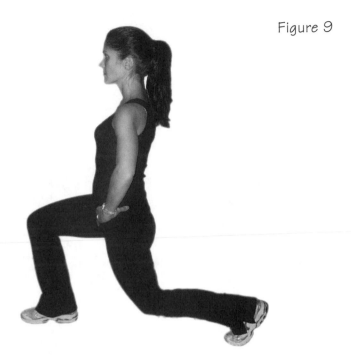

Figure 9

Lunges

Following our shoulder workout, we are going to move on to legs! Lunges are great for firming up the **buttocks and thighs**!

To perform correctly, stand with your feet shoulder width apart and your hands on your hips. Tighten your abdominal muscles while pulling your pelvis forward and straighten the curve in your lower back.

Place your right foot in front of you and your left foot behind you, See fig. 9. It is important to keep your torso perpendicular to the ground, and then lower yourself until your left knee is bent. For those who would like an extra challenge, jump slightly off the ground and scissor your legs so when you land your legs will be in a reverse position from when you started. (Remember these challenges are only for the Intermediate and Advanced).

- Be sure to land with both knees bent and your weight on the heel of your front foot and the ball of your back foot.
- Repeat this movement for fifteen reps, alternating legs each time.

Upon completion, get back on stability ball and repeat the set of **shoulder presses** again, followed by fifteen reps of **lunges**.

Figures 10 and 11

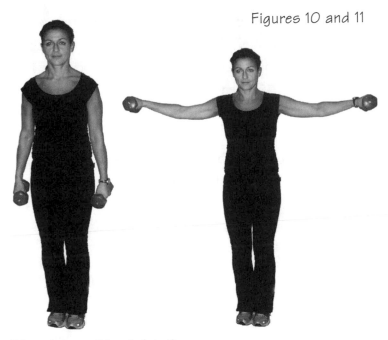

Shoulders/Upright Rows

Next, stand upright with your knees hip width apart and slightly bent.

With your light weights in hand and maintaining a slight bend in your elbows, raise the weights just above shoulder level. At the top of your movement your fingers should be pointed out and your thumbs pointing down. Keeping control of your movements, slowly lower the weights into your original position see fig. 10 & 11. Once fifteen reps have been executed, move on to perform **upright rows.**

To properly perform the upright rows, once again position yourself standing up with feet shoulder width apart. Slightly bending your knees, grasp the weights in your hands. Holding the weights, your palms should be facing in towards your body in front of your thighs.

Pull upward with the dumbbells to the front of your shoulders, but make sure to keep your elbows in tight against your body, see fig 12. Allow your wrists to flex as you raise the weight upward. Once you reach the height of your chin, slowly begin to lower back to original position.

Repeat this motion fifteen times.

Figure 12

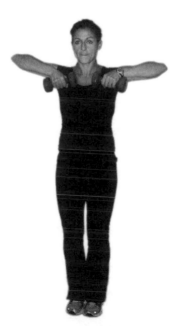

Reverse Flies

Next we will be moving on to **reverse flies.**

This exercise can be executed using the stability ball or by simply bending your body forward in the position of the number seven.

Let me first discuss how to execute this exercise with the stability ball. Begin this exercise by balancing your body at the center of the ball with your legs straight and toes to the floor. Hold your weights (for this exercise I recommend using your light weights as a correct body position & form is critical) to the right and left of the ball, underneath your shoulders with your arms extended.

- Bend over in the 7 position
- Raise your arms to your sides and bring the weights up to shoulder height. Try to keep your arms as straight as possible while making sure you don't lock your elbows.
  - Slowly lower the weights back to your original position, and complete set of fifteen reps.
  - The movements for this exercise in standing position are the same; simply begin it bent over in the seven position, with your knees slightly bent. Next begin to raise your arms toward shoulder height and then return back to original position.

Upon completion repeat **lateral lifts, upright rows, and reverse flies** for another fifteen rep set each.

Ball Chest Press

The next exercise we will be discussing is the **ball chest press**. See fig 13, 14 & 15.

Begin by sitting on the stability ball. Lying on the ball and placing your mid back on it, place your ankles directly under your bent knees. Lift your hips to the sky, and grab a weight in each hand.

Figure 13

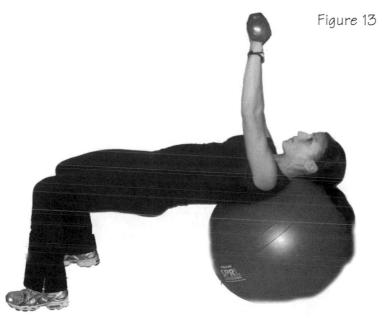

Figure 14

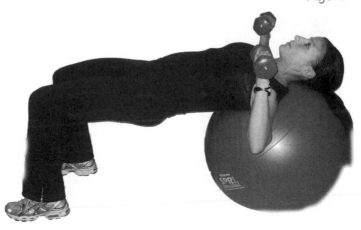

Figure 15

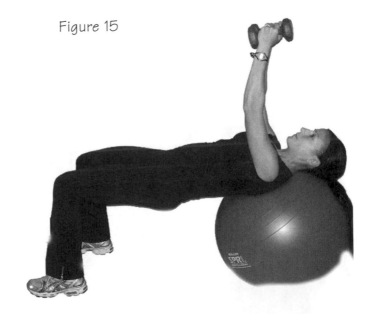

Lift the dumbbells up to the sky by extending your arms upward. Make sure you don't lock out your elbows! Pause once you reach full extension and hold for one second. Next, slowly lower the weight back to your original position. If you feel you are losing control of your body you are using the wrong weight and should switch to a lighter one. Ideally, you want to use only your chest and arm muscles to lift the weight.

Once you complete your set of fifteen reps, you are going to remain in the same position to complete another set of fifteen **stability ball chest flies.**

With your weights in hands, arms at your sides, and palms facing each other, slowly begin to lift the weights up over your ribcage. At the peak of the exercise your two weights will meet over the center of your chest. Make sure you don't lock your elbows! Hold at the peak for a moment, and then slowly lower the weights back to the original position. Do 15 reps. Upon completion combine both presses and flys for 10 reps. Immediately following exercise get into **push up position** (see fig. 3 & 4) for 15 reps.

Figure 17

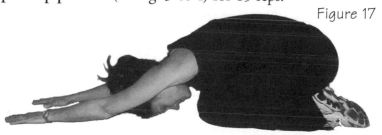

Repeat sets again for both chest **presses and flies**, 15 reps and 10 when combined.

At this point we are going to put the ball away for the time being and repeat another set of pushups. Remember to keep abs tight throughout! After your last pushup, get down into a yoga child's pose, (see fig. 17) and hold it for thirty seconds. To execute this position correctly, begin by getting down onto your knees and leaning your chest forward to the ground. Sit your hips back into your heels and extend your arms forward. Rest your forehead on the floor. Breathe in and relax your neck, face, and shoulders. Be sure to keep your arms stretched and your fingers spread.

This exercise relieves tension in the neck, shoulders, and thoracic spine, while also reducing menstrual pain!

Plank Pose

From the child's pose we are going to move up into the plank pose, see fig. 16. The benefits of this pose are that it strengthens your arms and spine, as well as your core muscles or abs, while preparing your body for more challenging arm balances.

Begin by drawing your torso forward until your shoulders are over your wrists and your whole body is in one straight line. This pose is very similar to the position you would be in before beginning your pushup exercise.

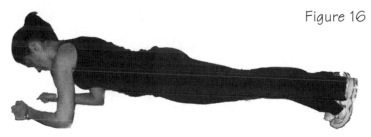

Figure 16

- Press your forearms and hands down firmly, while making sure you do not let your chest sink, and press back through your heels. Tighten your abs by sucking your naval into your spine.
- Keep your neck in line with your spine and broaden your shoulder blades.
- Hold this pose for thirty seconds.
- After the thirty seconds, drop your knees back into the child's pose for another thirty seconds and then repeat the plank pose.

Ab Workout

Next, we are going to begin our **ab workout!**

Our first exercise will be the **bicycle ab exercise.** To begin, lie face up on the floor and place your fingers behind your head.

- Bring your right knee in toward your chest while lifting your head and shoulder blades slightly off of the ground, making sure to keep your neck straight.

- Next, straighten your left leg outward to about a forty-five degree angle, while simultaneously shifting your upper body to the right, bringing your left elbow towards your right knee.

Switch sides so that you now will be bringing your right elbow towards your left knee, and continue alternating sides slowly in a cycling motion for thirty reps, which will be a total of fifteen reps per leg. For optimal results it is important that you conduct this exercise slowly in order to fully bring your muscles to the point of fatigue. The slower the movement the more results you will see.

Make sure you do not allow the extended leg to touch the floor; the lower you get it to the floor without touching it will intensify the stress on your abs!

Repeat for two sets.

Crunches

Next, we're going to move on to **crunches**, which we will be completing in two sets of twenty-five reps.

- To begin remain on the floor lying on your back, bend your knees keeping your feet on the floor and placing your hands behind your head or across your chest.

- Pull your belly button towards your spine and slowly contract your abdominals, bringing your shoulder blades about one or two inches off of the floor.
- Bring your knees in towards your chest at the same time as you lift your upper body off the floor, making sure you exhale as you come up. Be sure to keep your neck straight with your chin pointed upward.
- Hold the pose at the top of the movement for a few seconds, while continuing your breathing.
- Slowly lower your back and knees down, but don't completely relax, as you want to maintain stress on your abs.

9

Welcome to the Gym

The Beginner

Now, for the true beginner who has never worked out before, you may want to stay away from the weights for *only* the first week. You are not going to get off that easy because you are a virgin to the fitness world! For our first week we will be focusing on doing calorie burning cardio by walking! Yes, walking...*rapido,* that is! Each day we will gradually be increasing the time on the treadmill or outdoor walk from ten minutes our first day out to thirty minutes by the seventh day.

Vamonos...

We will be rating the intensity of our walks on a scale of 1to10, with 1 being slow and deliberate, and 10 being fast and intense! You will be using cardio to burn calories and blast your fat away! Listen to your heart rate and watch your sweat drip, because you will be sweating by the end of these walks!

- 3-4 intensity level Easy enough that you can sing
- 5-6 intensity level Moderate enough that you can talk and hold a conversation
- 7-8 intensity level Brisk enough that you can hold a conversation but rather not.

Day One—Let's begin by walking at a 3to 4 intensity level, for ten to fifteen minutes. You should be able to sing along to *"La Vida Loca!"*

Day Two—Walk fifteen to eighteen minutes at a moderate pace with no less than an intensity level of 4.

Day Three—Walk eighteen to twenty minutes at moderate pace while hitting an intensity level of between 5 to 6, but you should still be able to speak freely without gasping for breath in between words.

Day Four—Walk twenty to twenty-three minutes at moderate pace once again, but push yourself to a solid level 6 in intensity.

Day Five—Walk twenty-three to twenty-five minutes at moderate to intense pace, 7 to 8 level while gradually increasing your speed. Now you should still be able to talk, but I recommend you don't so you can focus on your breathing. As your speed increases, breathing is essential to prevent cramping.

Day Six—Walk twenty-five to twenty-eight minutes moderate to intense, reaching a level 8 intensity; here you will notice your increase in heart rate and sweating. Keep it up!

Day Seven—Walk thirty minutes at intense speed, maintaining a level 8 intensity. After completing the speed walk, walk for a few minutes at a slow to moderate speed, 3-4 intensity, to allow yourself to cool down. By doing so you allow your heart, lungs, and blood flow to gradually return to normal. This decreases strain on your heart and can prevent muscle strain and soreness.

Once you have completed week one and you are still not comfortable moving on to the first routine, rest your body for one day and repeat your day seven walk 3-4 times a week, while adding the dips, pushups, and abs workout from the first routine at the end of your workout. Complete with three sets of fifteen reps. Remember, the weight segment is as crucial as the cardio is in being the key to jump-starting your weight loss and new lifestyle.

Completo…lo isiste!!

Don't you feel GREAT!! Tired, pumped up, and GREAT! Stick to the program and I guarantee you will see results. But don't despair; this is a life changing, life altering state of mind which doesn't happen overnight. You have to wholehearted-ly commit to the new you, and you *will* love the person you see in the mirror as well as the one you feel deep inside. Ladies, it's so important to fully grasp that it doesn't matter what you look like on the outside if you don't like who you are inside. The complete package is the gift to a brilliant life in everything you do and for everyone you touch.

Part 3
Las Recetas
The Recipes

Barbara has changed my life! I can eat arroz con frijoles and not feel guilty! My body and most importantly attitude has never been better! I never thought it could be possible until I met her. Luckily I did!

—Jorge

10
"Exquisito!"
Platos Típicos Latinos

There are so many great dishes you can still enjoy while adding a healthy twist. You would be amazed and pleasantly surprised to find you don't have to cut out the things you love. Although the purpose of this book is to serve as a guide to fitness, and not be a cookbook, I have included a few of my favorite recipes I'd like to share with you in getting you started on the right track.

The following dishes could be eaten alone, with brown rice, wheat crackers, or your occasional *arroz blanco o galletas...buen aprovecho, salud.*

Pure de Boniato
Sweet Potato Mash

4 medium sweet potatoes peeled
1 tbsp of smart balance light butter
¼ cup of skim/low fat milk
Salt & Pepper to taste

Cut potatoes in halves and place in medium sauce pan, cover with water and add a pinch of salt. Bring to a boil and cook until tender. Remove potatoes and mash adding remaining ingredients. Serve!

Sweet potatoes are delicious and very healthy!! I love them with just about anything from Filet Mignon to Filet of Sole add sautéed mushrooms or vegetable of your choice and you will have an amazingly healthy delicious experience! Remember experimenting in the kitchen by tasting as you go along is the key to a happier and healthier you!

Buen Aprovecho!

Frijoles Negros
Black Beans

two tbsp. of EVOO
one tsp. oregano
one fifteen-oz. can of black beans in its water
one tsp. cumin
one half cup of chopped onion
one tsp. Goya adobo
one quarter cup of chopped green pepper
one tbsp. cooking dry white wine
two minced garlic cloves
dash of salt
Three quarters cup of water from can

In a medium-sized saucepan heat oil over medium heat, adding onion, pepper, and garlic. When tender stir in beans, water, oregano, cumin, adobo, wine, & salt. Cover and bring to a boil. Reduce heat to low and simmer for about ten minutes.

Serves four

Frijoles Colorado Con Puerco
Red Kidney Beans with Tenderloin of Pork

two tbsp. of EVOO

one quarter tsp. oregano

one fifteen-oz. can of red kidney beans with water

one quarter tsp. cumin

one half cup of chopped tenderloin of pork

one tsp. Goya adobo

one half cup of chopped onion

three quarters cup water from can

one half cup of chopped green pepper

two minced garlic cloves

In a medium-sized saucepan heat your oil with garlic, onion, pepper, and pork. Cover and cook over medium heat for ten minutes or until pork is cooked. Slowly stir in beans, tomato sauce, oregano, cumin, adobo, and water. Bring to a boil and then simmer for another ten minutes.

Serves four

Tostones con Mojo
Fried Plantains with Garlic Sauce

A favorite addition to any Latin dish

4 green plantains
1 cup vegetable or corn oil (your preference)
Salt to black pepper to taste
1 chopped garlic clove
¼ cup of sour orange juice (naranja agria)

Peel plantains and cut in pieces of about one inch thick. Heat ¾ cup of oil in a heavy skillet and fry plantains for about 5 minutes or until golden brown. Remove sliced plantains and place on cutting board or dish. Press with paper towel, foil, or spatula to flatten, sprinkle with salt and return to skillet with hot oil until crisp. Remove tostones from skillet and place on dish covered with paper towel. Season with salt and pepper.

Meanwhile, in a small dish, whisk garlic, remaining oil, and orange juice. Sprinkle over tostones and serve!

Tostones Rellenos
Stuffed Plantains

Definitely one of my favorites!!! You can stuff tostones with *picadillo de carne, picadillo de pavo, picadillo de pollo,* shrimp, crabmeat, anything! Ground beef, ground chicken, or ground turkey, anything! *Exquisito!* Delish!

You will use the same recipe from the *Tostones with Mojo* without the *mojo.* Along with the *Picadillo de Truiji,* my fathers recipe. However you can add anything.

The only difference to this dish is that when you remove the tostones from the skillet, you do not flatten them with the spatula, instead you get yourself a shot glass to make an indentation in its middle so that it looks like a cup. Place cupped *tostones* in a baking dish, preheat oven to 350 degrees and fill each one with your favorite filling which you have already prepared and is on the side. Bake for 8 minutes, remove and let cool. If you want to spice it up a notch sprinkle a dash of hot sauce! *Caliente!*

Ensalada de Aguacate con Tomate
Avocado& Tomato Salad

1 large Florida Avocado or two Haas
½ cup chopped cilantro
1 diced medium tomato
¼ cup chopped basil
1 diced red onion
Salt & Pepper to Taste
¼ cup EVOO & White wine vinegar

Slice the avocado from top to bottom in quarters, remove skin and chop in about 1 inch pieces. Combine the diced tomato and red onion in a small bowl. Make the dressing by whisking together the EVOO, vinegar, basil, salt and pepper. Toss all ingredients together gently, avocados are very delicate. Place on serving dish and garnish with cilantro.

Serves three

You can have this dish as a side salad or as a topping over fresh grilled fish such as Tilapia.
One of my favorites and very easy to make.

Ensalada de Garbanzos
Chick Pea Salad

1 15 oz can of chick peas drained
¼ cup EVOO
1 medium tomato diced
¼ cup lime juice
1 red onion diced
¼ cup chopped cilantro
1 cup diced red bell pepper
¼ cup chopped basil & thyme
Salt & Pepper to taste

Whisk EVOO, lime juice, basil, thyme, salt & pepper and set aside. Drain and rinse chick peas and toss with tomato, onion, and pepper. Mix all ingredients together and sprinkle with chopped cilantro. Chill and serve.

Serves four

Tortilla Española
Spanish Tortilla

4 large potatoes, peeled and thinly sliced
1 cup EVOO
8 egg whites
Salt & Pepper to taste
1 egg yolk
1 large onion thinly sliced

In a large skillet heat the oil over medium heat. Add onions and potatoes, stirring occasionally so that they don't stick until they are soft. Remove from the skillet drain the oil and set aside. Reserve about 3 tbsp. of the EVOO. In a large bowl beat the eggs and mix in with the potatoes and onions. Add the 2 tbsp. of the oil back into the skillet over medium heat. When the pan is hot add the egg mixture and spread covering the full pan. Add the salt and pepper and shake the pan occasionally to prevent sticking. When the potatoes begin to brown and the tortilla begins to harden grab a plate and place it over the skillet to flip. Remove any pieces that may have stuck on the skillet, add the remaining tbsp of EVOO and slide the tortilla back onto the pan. Cover and let it sit over medium to low heat until it is firm. You may have to flip it one more time if necessary. Remove and enjoy!

Tortillas could be served for breakfast in wedges as well as in small squares as tapas for h'ordeuvres.

Six servings
Twelve tapas

Carnes
Beef, Pork and Poultry

We love beef in our home, but yes, we eat seafood and poultry in order to maintain our balanced nutrition; however, find me a Latin person who does not love a plate of *Picadillo* with just about anything. Not long ago, over a family gathering we discussed the many dishes one could make with *Picadillo*. The list is endless…so whether it's over a nice healthy salad or a plate of rice (brown or white) *picadillo* is a dish that will go a long way. Enjoy!

Picadillo a la Truji
Ground Beef a la Truji

one lb. lean ground beef*
one tsp. of golden mustard
one tbsp. of EVOO
dash of Worcestershire sauce
one half cup chopped onion
one tsp. Goya adobo
one quarter cup chopped green pepper
one tbsp. of cooking dry white wine
one minced garlic clove
two tbsp of pitted olives with pimientos
small can of tomato sauce & its juice w/garlic & onion

In a medium-sized skillet heat oil over medium heat adding garlic, onion & pepper until tender. Add beef, tomato sauce, adobo, mustard, Worcestershire sauce, & wine. Cover and cook for ten minutes stirring occasionally. When beef is fully cooked bring heat to low and add olives with pimientos and its juice. Stir and serve.

Serves four

The ground beef could also be substituted with ground turkey or ground chicken breast.

Bistec Empanizado
Breaded Steak

one lb. palomilla steak
one half tbsp. of salt
one half tbsp. of garlic powder
one cup of whole grain bread crumbs
one half tbsp. of Goya adobo
one quarter tbsp. of pepper
two eggs
one cup vegetable oil
one lime

The steaks should be thinly cut into about six pieces. Season them with the pepper, garlic and adobo and put aside. Beat the eggs with the salt. Place the steaks in the eggs and then the bread crumbs to fully cover each steak. Fry them in hot EVOO until fully cooked. Place a paper towel over a plate to allow the excess oil to drip off once removed from the skillet. Squeeze lime juice over steaks before serving.

Serves six

Bistec Encebollado
Steak with Onions

2 pounds of thinly sliced sirloin steak
¼ cup chopped cilantro
2 cups of sliced yellow onion
salt & pepper to taste
¼ cup EVOO
fresh lime juice
4 minced garlic cloves
Goya adobo
Cumin

Pound the steaks to about ¼ inch thickness, season and rub with salt, pepper, cumin, and adobo and set aside. Heat the EVOO in a large skillet and sauté onion briefly over medium heat until slightly tender and beginning to brown. Remove and set aside. Add the garlic to the skillet and sauté, add steak and cook. The steaks should take no more than 5 minutes since they are thin and will cook quickly. Remember to flip over on both sides to cook evenly. It shouldn't take no more than a minute or two on each side. It all depends on how you prefer your steaks, medium to well, etc. Right before you about to take them out bring the onion back for one last stir, enough to warm them and bring all flavors together. Remove, sprinkle with lime juice and cilantro and serve!

Serves four

Salsa Roja
Red Sauce

8oz can Tomato sauce w/garlic & onion
¼ cup dry red cooking wine
28 oz can whole peeled tomatoes w/basil
1 oz Goya capers
¼ cup EVOO
1 can Goya black olives
1/3 cup minced garlic
Salt & Pepper to taste
1 med yellow onion sliced in rounds
½ cup chopped cilantro

In a large skillet over low to medium heat add EVOO, garlic, & onion. When onion becomes tender and slightly browned add tomatoes and sauce. Mash tomatoes so that they are chopped into small pieces and its natural juices are combined. Stirring occasionally add the remaining ingredients, cover and let simmer so that all flavors infuse.

This sauce could be used with just about anything. You could add your favorite fresh filet of fish or mine such as sole or salmon. While it's simmering add the filet, cover and cook for about 5 minutes. I have added my pork tenderloin recipe for your enjoyment! Enjoy!

Chuleta en Salsa Roja
Pork Tenderloin in Red Sauce

Red sauce recipe and ingredients are necessary for this delicioso dish.

Add: 2 pork tenderloins about 2 lbs.
Goya Adobo
Salt & Pepper to taste

Trim off the skin and tissue from the tenderloins, rub with adobo, salt & pepper on both sides and set aside. While the red sauce is simmering, before adding the capers and olives, add the tenderloins to the skillet. Cover and cook each side for about 5 minutes each or until they are cooked through. Add the capers and olives and stir. Remove and garnish with cilantro.

Serves 2

Frijoles Colorado Con Puerco
Red Kidney Beans with Tenderloin of Pork

two tbsp. of EVOO

one quarter tsp. oregano

one fifteen-oz. can of red kidney beans with water

one quarter tsp. cumin

one half cup of chopped tenderloin of pork

 one tsp. Goya adobo

one half cup of chopped onion

three quarters cup water from can

one half cup of chopped green pepper

two minced garlic cloves

In a medium-sized saucepan heat your oil with garlic, onion, pepper, and pork. Cover and cook over medium heat for ten minutes or until pork is cooked. Slowly stir in beans, tomato sauce, oregano, cumin, adobo, and water. Bring to a boil and then simmer for another ten minutes.

Serves four

Ropa Vieja
Old Clothes (don't let the name fool you)

two lbs. skirt steak*
one can tomato sauce with onion and garlic
one third cup of EVOO
one tbsp. salt
one onion chopped
two tbsp. cilantro
two garlic cloves chopped
one tsp. cumin
one green pepper chopped
one bay leaf
one can red peppers *(pimiento morrones)*

In a saucepan bring salted water to a boil and cook steak over medium heat for about ten minutes or until fully cooked. Drain the water, let it cool and shred the beef. In a skillet heat the oil and add the onion, garlic, and pepper. Mix until tender, then add the tomato sauce, cumin, and bay leaf. Add the shredded beef and cook for another ten minutes stirring occasionally. Remove from heat, discard the bay leaf, and serve with the pimiento morrones and cilantro with salad or over rice.

Serves eight

*The skirt steak could also be substituted with chicken breast or turkey breast.

Bistec de Pollo a la Plancha
Grilled Chicken Breasts

4 chicken breast cutlets
¼ cup chopped cilantro
¼ cup chopped yellow onion
Cumin
¼ cup EVOO
Salt & Pepper to taste
Dash of Goya Adobo
¼ cup Goya Mojo Marinade

Season chicken with salt, pepper, adobo, & cumin. In a large skillet, sauté onion with EVOO over medium heat until it becomes tender and begins to brown. Remove onion and set aside. In same skillet keeping EVOO add chicken with Mojo Marinade. Cover and cook over medium heat until thoroughly cooked through. Do not overcook it should take no more than 8-10 minutes. Once cooked, remove chicken without liquid and drizzle with onion and cilantro.

Serves four

For an added touch make the black beans from earlier and serve over chicken! You will love it!! OR add the avocado salad, OR the mango salad over the chicken!!

Arroz con Pollo de Mami
Mami's Chicken with Yellow Rice

½ cup EVOO
1 can of asparagus
6 chicken breasts cut into chunks
2 packets of sazon Goya con azafran
2 chopped onions
1 cup dry white wine
3 minced garlic cloves
2 cups of light chicken broth
1 large diced green pepper
2 bay leaves
1 can of tomato sauce
salt and pepper to taste
1 can of fancy pimientos (morrones)
dash of cumin
1 can of petit pois (sweet peas)
3 cups of long grain rice washed

Season the chicken with the garlic, salt and pepper. Heat the oil
in a large roaster or stock pot adding chicken so that it browns
along with onion, pepper, cumin, sazon with azafran, bay leaves,
tomato sauce, white cooking wine, and chicken broth. Add the

rice to the pot along with the liquid of the fancy pimientos, sweet peas, and asparagus. Cook everything over low heat until the grain of rice is open and tender. Decorate your Arroz con Pollo with the pimientos, asparagus, and petit pois (I love that name and you will love the dish!!)

Eight servings

Pescado
Seafood

Camarones al Ajillo
Shrimp in Garlic Sauce

2 lbs. medium cooked shrimp
pinch of oregano
½ cup EVOO
pinch of parsley
15 Garlic cloves crushed
salt & pepper to taste
3 tbsp dry white cooking wine
pinch of cilantro for garnish
2 limes juiced

In a large frying pan sauté garlic in oil until golden brown. Add shrimp and remaining ingredients and cook over medium heat for about 10 minutes stirring and blending occasionally. Garnish with cilantro and serve. This dish is amazing with any type of rice, or my favorite sweet potato mash.

Pescado en Salsa Verde
Filet of Fish in "Salsa Verde"

1 ½ lbs. of Sole, Tilapia, or any boneless filet of your favorite white fish

Salsa verde:
1 garlic clove
1 tsp salt
1 cup EVOO
1 tsp Goya Adobo
1 medium onion
2 tbsp of white wine vinegar
1 cup of parsley
½ cup dry white cooking wine

Blend together all the ingredients of salsa in a food processor. Place fish in a pan over medium heat and cover with salsa. When the salsa starts to boil cover the pan, lower heat to low and let cook for about 10 to 15 minutes until fish is white and flakey.

6 servings...enjoy!

Garbanzos Con Bacalao
Chickpeas with Codfish

one lb. of chickpeas (garbanzos)
one can of tomato sauce w/garlic and onion
one lb. of codfish (no bones)
one half cup of EVOO (extra virgin olive oil)
one can of fancy pimientos
one large onion chopped
one quarter cup of dry white cooking wine
two garlic cloves chopped
dash of salt
one large green pepper chopped
one third cup of parsley chopped

Soak the chickpeas with the codfish for two to three hours. Remove the water and separate the chickpeas from the fish. Cover the garbanzos with approx. four cups of water over medium flame until the beans soften which should take about one hour, however, longer if necessary. When the beans are soft, in a frying pan heat the EVOO and add the onion and pepper until tender, then add the garlic. Let fry for a few minutes. Add the tomato sauce, fancy pimientos with the water, parsley and white wine. Bring all to a boil in a large pot with the fish, garbanzos softened and one cup of its water. Cook all on low heat for about one half hour. The amount of salt varies since cod is salty by nature.

Eight servings

Tilapia a la Plancha
Grilled Tilapia

4 filets of Tilapia
¼ cup chopped parsley
¼ cup Lemon Juice
Salt & Pepper to taste
1 tbs. Smart Balance Light Butter

In a large skillet melt butter over medium heat. Place fish add lemon juice and cover. Bring heat to low and cook for about 5 minutes or until fish is flaky. Once done add parsley, salt and pepper and serve. Garnish with mango salsa or avocado salad or simply enjoy alone with salad or vegetable of your choice.

Serves four

Postre
Dessert

Flan de Lola
Lola's Flan

Since we love sweets and can't live without them I have enticed you with one of my favorites from Blanca's kitchen, her mother's healthy alternative to our favorite…the Flan!

1 eggland egg
½ bar of fat free cream cheese
4 egg whites
1 cup of sugar
1 can evaporated fat free milk
1 can fat free condensed milk

In a small saucepan over low heat add sugar stirring occasionally until it caramelizes. Transfer the caramelized sugar onto a 10 inch baking pan and evenly spread throughout the bottom of the pan. Place it aside to cool off.

Preheat oven to 350

Blend remaining ingredients in a blender until well mixed. Once sugar is cool add blended mixture into the baking pan. Cover with aluminum foil, place in a "*baño Maria*"* and bake for 1 hour or until knife inserted in the middle comes out clean. Once baked remove from oven and "*baño*

Maria", set aside and let cool. Place in refrigerator overnight. The following day remove it from the baking pan by gently removing it from the edges with a knife, place your serving dish on top covering the baking pan and flip. It's ready to serve! My mouth waters just thinking about it!! A perfect ending to a great meal!

*Baño Maria is when you place one dish into another with water in it. In this case you will fill a pan 1/3 its way with water and place the baking dish inside making sure the water does not spill into it. You are cooking with the heated water and oven.

Translation Please...
A Glossary of Spanish Terms
in Order of Appearance

"Barbara por Atras" – a persons name, and also defined as
    Amazing. Complete term "Amazing from Behind"

"Que linda con su culo parado" – "How adorable with her
    cute puffy ass"

Piropos – compliments.

Caderas – hips

Comida Criolla – creole dishes

"Con orgullo te presento…." – "With pride I present…"

"…por que somos, y gracias a Dios…" – "Because we are
    and thank God we will continue to be, Amazing from
    Behind, Amazing from the Front, and Amazing from
    Inside."

"…la vida es un carnival, hay que vivir cantando…" –
    "…life is a carnival, you have to live singing…there is no
    need to cry…the sorrows will go away singing…"

Arroz con Frijoles – rice and beans

Tostones Rellenos – stuffed plantains

Cortadito – miniature café con leche, espresso with steamed
    milk.

"Soy Latina..." – "I am a Latin woman"

Azucar! – sugar, "Spice!" A word made popular by the leg-
    endary Cuban artist Celia Cruz

Pastelitos – pastries

"Santa Barbara…santa por adelante y barbara por atrás..."
    – "Saint Barbara…heavenly from the front, amazing
    from behind..."

"Pues aqui vamos" – "Well here we go"

"Que rica estas" – "You are so delicious"

"Estas por la maseta" – "You are hard and hot"

"Que nalgas mas buenas tienes" – "What a great ass
    you have"

"Si cocina como caminas…." – "If you cook like you walk
    I'd eat all the scraps"

Natilla con dulce de leche – a dessert made of vanilla
    custard and sweet milk

"Para seguir la tradicion y orgullo…" - "To continue the tra-
    dition and pride of having a great body"

"Te mandaría para el carajo" – I'd send you to hell

Masita de puerco con arroz y platano maduros – fried pork
    with rice and fried plantains

Chancleta – slipper

"...mami, y papi donde estes..." – "...mom, and dad wher-
    ever you may be, thank you again."

"La dieta se empieza mañana" – "The diet starts tomorrow"

"Eso no engorda" – "That isn't fattening"

"Un dia no hace nada" – "One day doesn't do anything"

"Todo lo Exagerado es Malo" – "All types of excessive behav-
    ior, exaggerations, are bad"

"Pero lo somo" – "But we are"

"Somo exajerado de naturaleza" – "It is in our nature to
    exaggerate"

Arroz Integral – brown rice

"El bistecito" – the steak

"cuando yo vivía en Cuba" – "when I lived in Cuba"

Mojitos – classic Cuban cocktail made of rum with sugar and
    mint

Tapas – Spanish savory snacks

"y que se repite" – "and may it be repeated"

"Tenemos Caderas" – "We have Hips"

"Tenemos Murlos" – "We have Thighs"

"Tenemos Nalgas" – "We have an Ass"

"Tenemos Curvas" – "We have Curves"

"Tenemos Tetas" – "We have Tits"

"Tenemos Sangre" – "We have Blood/ Spice"

"Somos Latinas!!!" – "We are Latin Woman!!!"

"A Comer" – "to eat"

Arroz con frijoles – rice and beans

Arroz con huevo frito – rice with egg sunny side up

Arroz con sardinas – rice with sardines

Arroz con gandules – rice with a type of bean

Arroz con salchichas – rice with sausages

Arroz con vegetales – rice with vegetables

Arroz con leche – rice with milk

Arepa – a corn based bread

Novela – Spanish soap opera

Congris – white rice with black beans cooked together browning the rice

Pan con mantequilla – toasted bread with butter

"Todo con moderación no solo en la comida…" – "Everything within moderation not only in the kitchen but in every aspect f life."

"Porque gracias a Dios lo tenemos…" – "Because thank God we have it, the "fever", the blood, the love of being a Latin woman!"

"La Tortura" – "The Torture"

"A comenzar la tortura" – "To begin the torture"

"No te desesperes" – "Don't despair"

Rapido – fast

Vamonos – Let's go

"Completo…lo isiste!!" – "Complete…you did it!

"Exquisito." – "exquisite"

"Platos Tipicos Latinos" – "Typical Latin Dishes"

Galletas – crackers

"Buen aprovecho, salud" – "Enjoy, cheers"

Picadillo de Carne – ground beef

Picadillo de Pavo – ground turkey

Picadillo de Pollo – ground chicken

Caliente – hot

Truji – short for Trujillo, my maiden name and Dad's last name. What all his loved ones called him.

Arroz con Pollo de Mami – My mom's chicken with yellow rice

Lola – short for Dolores Blanca's mom

"Bano Maria" – "Maria's Bath" Cooking something in its pan with the heated water from the other pan its sitting in. Don't ask…your guess is as good as mine.

Gracias…Thank you…Cheers…Salud!